Jean-Claude Dubost

T hey're asleep. All of them. Or at least they seem to be. The baby lying on the donkey in the middle of a herd in Niger, the woman dozing on straw in Bali, the couple lying in a field in England, the man slumped in a chair in Hong Kong all radiate a feeling of restfulness, sometimes of torpor. By bringing them together, this book is tinged with a surprising mood, for although these dozing faces give rise to familiar impressions, each one of them tells us a different story. The mix of stories, the photographer's eye and our own individual experiences are what make the theme so rich. By seeking to capture the essentials of a scene in a 'decisive instant', the photographers have caught fleeting moments of sleep in their greatest variety.

What is most striking about these photographs is the subject matter's diversity. What do have in common two clarinet players sitting in a room, one of them with a hat pushed down over his face, the other with his head in his arms, and a satin-skinned woman lying in a park, her eyes closed, looking as if she were sunbathing? Their slumber tells us two very different things. In the first case, it expresses the weariness of labor or of waiting. In the second it evokes relaxation. The clarinet players seem to be waiting for a concert to start or resting after their performance. Perhaps they are tired after a long trip. The woman appears to be enjoying a good dose of summer sunshine on vacation.

In some instances, the variety of places and states of sleep becomes ambiguous. The picture can evoke refreshing slumber or, on the contrary, a fitful, anxiety-ridden sleep, close to lethargy. The man lying in the grass photographed by Henri Cartier-Bresson could be relaxing – or in a drunken stupor. The photographs' indefinite character makes various interpretations possible. We don't know whether these people are taking a nap, sleeping it off after a bout of drinking, or relaxing. The myriad of possible perspectives and interpretations can be found in the picture of the Madrid lottery-ticket vendor. She's slumped in a chair on the street against a wall, covering her face and hands with a sheet of newspaper. Then there's the naked woman lying lustfully on a bed of white sheets, a stole casually tossed over her thighs. And what about the mother carrying her child in her arms sitting on a sidewalk in Hong Kong, her eyes closed and her mouth open? Is she begging, praying or trying to enjoy a breath of fresh air in the stifling afternoon heat?

These pictures are contradictory and complementary at the same time. They show us the richness of the situations captured and possible ways of interpreting them. From county to city, this book takes us through the different worlds of sleep and also revives feelings and memories. A baby gone beddy-bye, a soldier resting after battle, a worker dozing, a homeless person slumbering, a merry-maker sleeping it off and every kind of nap are seen through the profoundly human eyes of Magnum photographers.

ls dorment. Tous. Ou du moins en ont-ils l'air. Ce bébé couché sur un âne au milieu d'un troupeau au Niger, cette femme endormie dans la paille à Bali, ce couple allongé dans un champ en Angleterre, cet homme affalé sur sa chaise à Hong Kong... Tous dégagent la même sensation de repos, parfois de torpeur. En les réunissant, le livre se teinte d'une atmosphère étonnante, car même si l'on retrouve dans ces visages assoupis des impressions familières, chacun d'entre eux nous raconte une histoire différente. Or, c'est ce mélange de leurs histoires, de celle du photographe et de la nôtre qui crée la richesse d'un tel thème. En cherchant à capter l'essentiel d'une scène dans un « instant décisif », les photographes ont su prendre au vol des bribes de vie dans ces instants de sommeil saisissants, et ils nous les restituent dans leur plus grande variété.

En effet, ce qui frappe avant tout, c'est la diversité du sujet même : quoi de commun entre ces deux clarinettistes assis dans une salle, l'un le chapeau rabattu sur son visage penché en avant et l'autre la tête dans ses bras, et cette femme allongée dans un parc, le visage satiné, les yeux plissés, semblant prendre un bain de soleil ? Leur sommeil nous dit deux choses très différentes : dans un cas, il exprime la fatigue du labeur ou de l'attente, dans l'autre, il évoque la détente des loisirs. Tandis que les premiers semblent attendre l'heure du concert ou bien se reposer après la prestation, fatigués peut-être du long voyage menant à ces Rencontres internationales de la clarinette en France, la deuxième a l'air de profiter d'un rayon de soleil estival et vacancier.

Cette diversité des lieux et des états du sommeil devient ambiguïté dans certains cas : l'image du dormeur peut évoquer la sieste réparatrice ou, au contraire, un sommeil inquiétant, proche de la léthargie : cet homme couché dans l'herbe, photographié par Henri Cartier-Bresson, peut aussi bien passer pour quelqu'un qui se délasse que pour un individu assommé par l'alcool. Le caractère indéfini de certaines photos suscite des interprétations diverses : on ne sait plus si ces gens dorment, cuvent leur vin, se détendent...

Cette multiplicité des regards et des lectures possibles se retrouve par exemple dans la photo de cette vendeuse madrilène de billets de loterie, campée sur une chaise dans la rue, contre un mur, qui se cache le visage et les mains sous une feuille de journal... De même, plusieurs réflexions s'imposent au regard de cette autre femme, couchée sur un lit de draps blancs, dénudée et dans une pose lascive, une étole négligemment jetée sur ses cuisses. Et cette mère portant son enfant dans les bras, assise sur un trottoir de Hong Kong, les yeux fermés et la bouche ouverte ? Mendie-t-elle, prie-t-elle ou tente-t-elle de profiter d'un souffle de fraîcheur dans la touffeur de l'après-midi ?

À la fois contradictoires et complémentaires, ces images nous montrent la richesse des situations saisies et des lectures possibles. De la campagne à la ville, ce livre nous promène ainsi à travers les horizons divers du sommeil, en même temps qu'il nous rappelle des émotions, des souvenirs. Dodo du bébé, repos du guerrier, répit du travailleur, sommeil du sans-abri, abandon de l'éméché, la sieste dans ses états tous vue par le regard profondément humain des photographes de Magnum.

Sleep ▪ *Sommeil* ▪ Der Schlaf

Photographs of Magnum Photos • *Photographies de Magnum Photos* • **Fotografien von Magnum Photos**

Editor: Jean-Claude Dubost
Desk Editor: Caroline Broué
Graphic design: Véronique Rossi
Iconographic and artistic coordination at Magnum Photos:
Marie-Christine Biebuyck and Agnès Sire,
assisted by Philippe Devernay, Marta Campos and Inessa Quenum
English translation: Glenn Naumovitz
Photoengraving: Litho Service T. Zamboni, Verona

© FINEST SA / EDITIONS PIERRE TERRAIL, Paris, 1998
The Art Book Subsidiary of BAYARD PRESSE SA
Magnum Photos, Paris, 1998
ISBN 2-87939-196-2
English edition: © 1998
Publication number: 237
Printed in Italy.

Direction éditoriale : Jean-Claude Dubost
Assistante éditoriale : Caroline Broué
Conception et réalisation graphique : Véronique Rossi
Direction iconographique et artistique à Magnum Photos :
Marie-Christine Biebuyck et Agnès Sire,
assistées de Philippe Devernay, Marta Campos et Inessa Quenum
Traduction anglaise : Glenn Naumovitz
Traduction allemande : Inge Hanneforth
Photogravure : Litho Service T. Zamboni, Vérone

© FINEST SA / ÉDITIONS PIERRE TERRAIL, Paris, 1998
La filiale Livres d'art de BAYARD PRESSE SA
Magnum Photos, Paris, 1998
ISBN 2-87939-183-0
N° d'éditeur : 237
Dépôt légal : octobre 1998
Imprimé en Italie.

Verlegerische Leitung: Jean-Claude Dubost
Verantwortlich für die Ausgabe: Caroline Broué
Buchgestaltung: Véronique Rossi
Bildredaktion und gragische Gestaltung für Magnum Photos:
Marie-Christine Biebuyck, Agnès Sire;
Assistenten: Philippe Devernay, Marta Campos, Inessa Quenum
Deutsche Übersetzung: Inge Hanneforth
Farblithos: Litho Service T. Zamboni, Verona

© FINEST SA / EDITIONS PIERRE TERRAIL, Paris, 1998
Der Bereich Kunstbücher von BAYARD PRESSE SA
Magnum Photos, Paris, 1998
ISBN 2-87939-196-2
Deutsche Ausgabe: © 1998
Verlegernummer: 237
Printed in Italy.

Sie schlafen. Alle. Zumindest sieht es so aus. Das inmitten einer Herde auf einen Esel gebettete Baby im Niger, die im Stroh eingeschlafene Frau in Bali, das auf einem Feld ruhende Paar in England, der auf seinem Stuhl zusammengesunkene Mann in Hongkong ... Sie alle verleihen den Eindruck, sich zu entspannen, manchmal aber auch, benommen zu sein. Das Besondere dieses Fotobandes ist seine große Diversifizität, denn selbst wenn man in diesen schlaftrunkenen Gesichtern oft einen bekannten Ausdruck bemerkt, so erzählt uns doch jeder seine Geschichte. Und die Mischung der Geschichte jedes einzelnen, die des Fotografen und unsere eigene ist es, die ein solches Thema besonders interessant macht. Indem die Fotografen versuchen, das Besondere eines bestimmten Augenblicks festzuhalten, zeigen sie jeweils winzige Lebensabschnitte dieser Schlafenden.

Die Vielfalt des Themas überrascht ganz besonders: Denn was verbindet zwei in einem Raum sitzende Klarinettisten - der eine den Hut ins Gesicht gezogen und nach vorn geneigt, der andere den Kopf in die Arme gebettet - mit der in einem Park ausgestreckten Frau mit seidig glänzendem Gesicht und leicht zusammengekniffen Augen, die ein Sonnenbad zu nehmen scheint? Der Schlaf all dieser Menschen drückt zwei sehr unterschiedliche Dinge aus: einerseits die Müdigkeit der Arbeit oder des Wartens, andererseits eher Entspannung und Freizeit. Während die ersten auf den Beginn des Konzerts zu warten oder sich nach dem Spielen und der langen Anreise zum internationalen Klarinettisten-Treffen in Frankreich auszuruhen scheinen, verleiht die Frau den Eindruck, die Sonne oder den Urlaub zu genießen. All diese unterschiedlichen Orte und Schlafzustände sind aber nicht immer eindeutig. Das Bild des Schläfers zeigt den erholsamen Mittagsschlaf, vielleicht aber auch den lethargischen Dämmerzustand: Den von Henri Cartier-Bresson fotografierten, im Gras liegenden Mann kann man beispielsweise für jemanden halten, der sich entspannt, aber auch für einen, der seinen Rausch ausschläft. Der unbestimmte Charakter einiger Fotos kann somit unterschiedlich interpretiert werden, denn man weiß nicht, ob diese Menschen ruhen, sich von dem Glas zuviel erholen oder sich ganz einfach entspannen ... All diese unterschiedlichen Auslegungen kommen besonders im Foto der Madrider Verkäuferin von Lotterielosen zum Ausdruck, die auf der Straße auf einem an die Wand gelehnten Stuhl sitzt und Gesicht und Hände unter einer Zeitung verbirgt. Auch die lasziv auf einem Bett mit weißen Laken hingestreckte nackte Frau, eine Stola lässig über die Beine geworfen, kann so und so gesehen werden. Und die Mutter mit ihrem Kind in den Armen, die, mit geschlossenen Augen und offenem Mund, auf einem Trottoir in Hongkong sitzt. Ist es eine Bettlerin, betet sie oder versucht sie, sich in der stickigen Mittagshitze etwas Kühle zu verschaffen?

Diese zugleich widersprüchlichen und sich ergänzenden Bilder zeigen uns die Fülle der festgehaltenen Situationen und der unterschiedlichen „Lesarten". Vom Land zur Stadt zeigt uns dieses Buch die zahlreichen Facetten des Schlafs und ruft beim Betrachten Gefühle und Erinnerungen hervor. Das schlummernde Baby, die Ruhepause des Kämpfers, das Nickerchen des Arbeiters, der Halbschlaf des Obdachlosen, der Dämmerzustand des Angetrunkenen und selbstverständlich der Mittagsschlaf: festgehalten von den größten Fotografen.

Jean-Claude Dubost

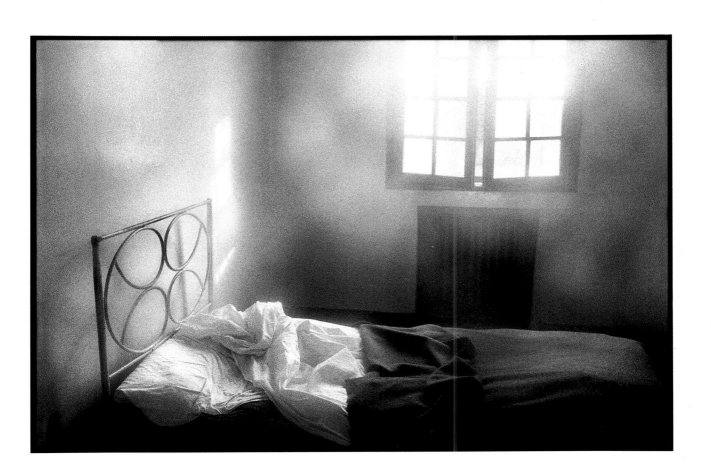

Raymond Depardon, Italy, *Italie,* Italien, 1979. | **7**

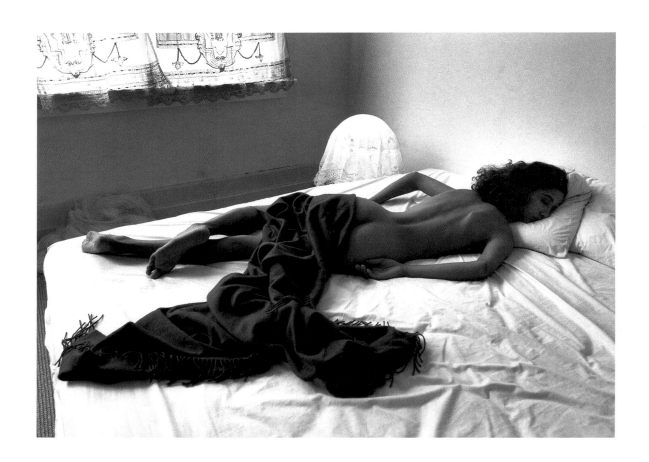

8 Ferdinando Scianna, Holland, *Pays-Bas,* Holland, 1990.

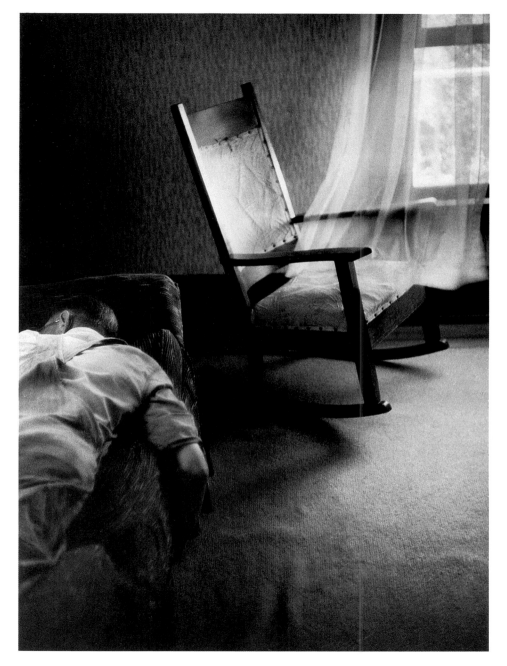

Erich Hartmann, USA, *États-Unis,* USA, 1956. **9**

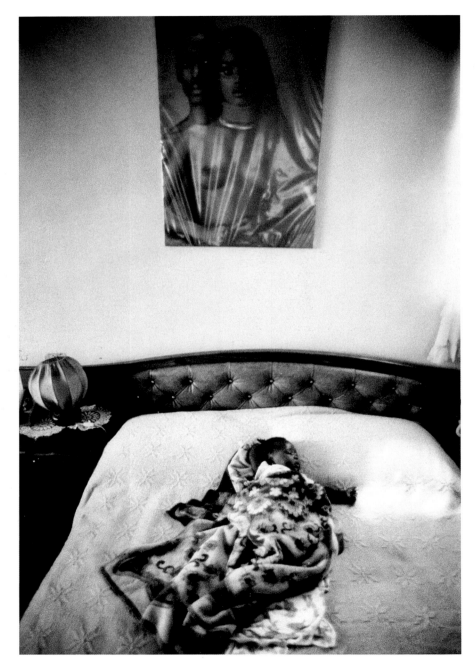

10 | Ian Berry, South Africa, *Afrique du Sud,* Sudafrika, 1984.

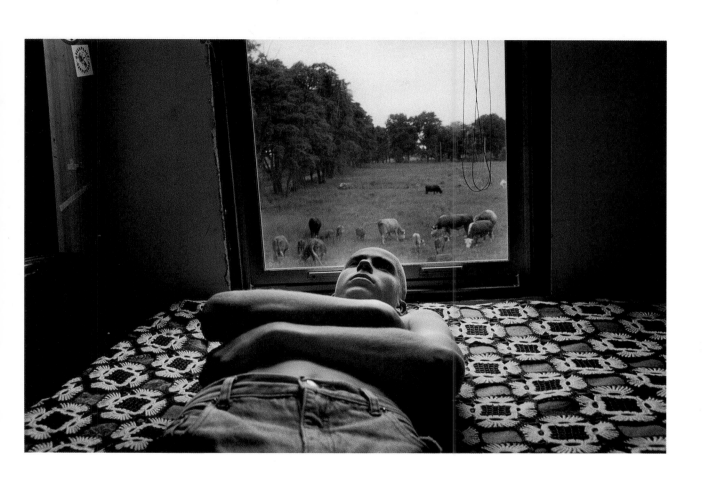

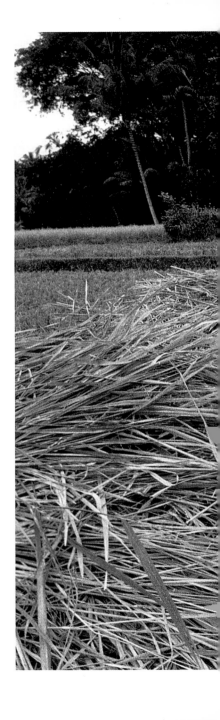

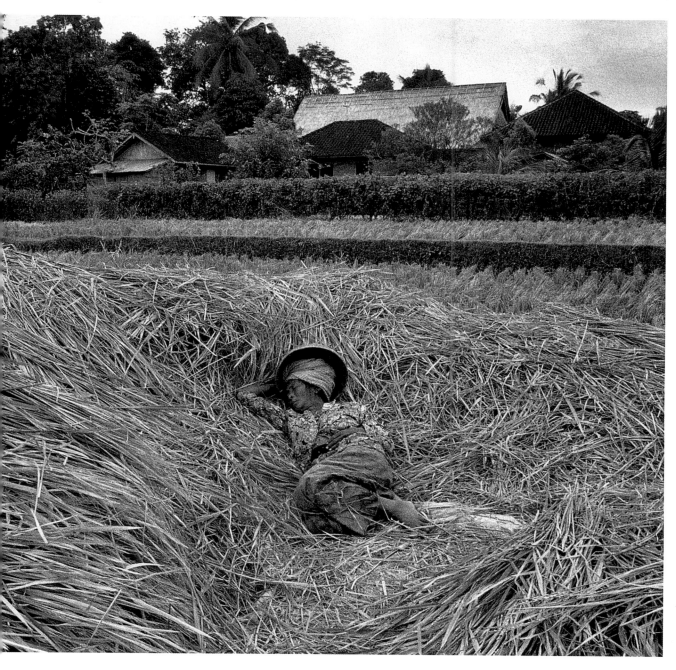

Ferdinando Scianna, Bali, *Bali,* Bali, 1989. **13**

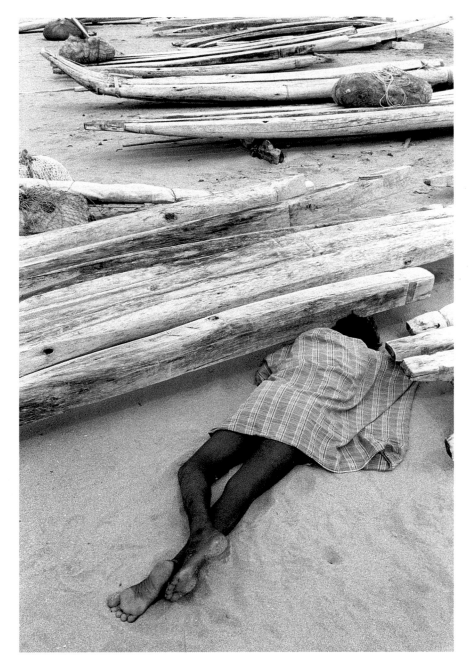

John Vink, India, *Inde,* Indien, 1987.

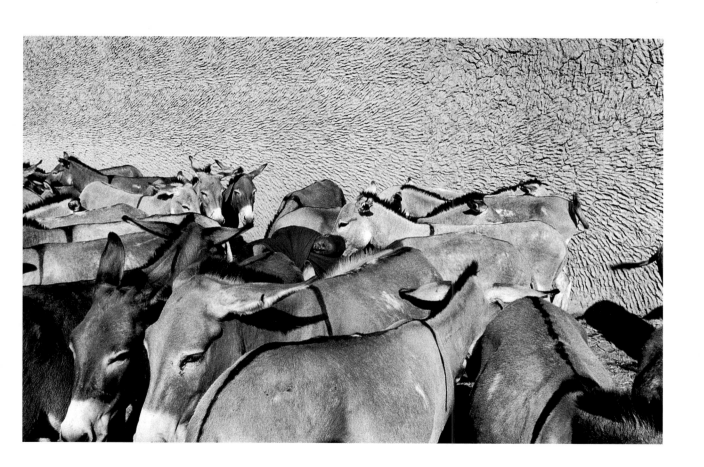

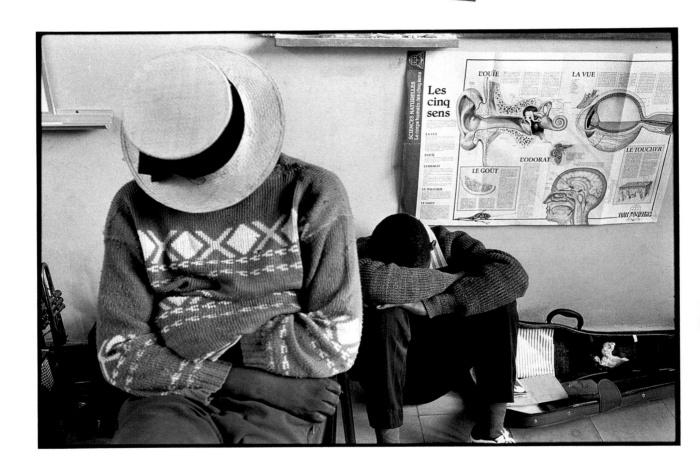

16 Guy Le Querrec, France, *France,* Frankreich, 1992.

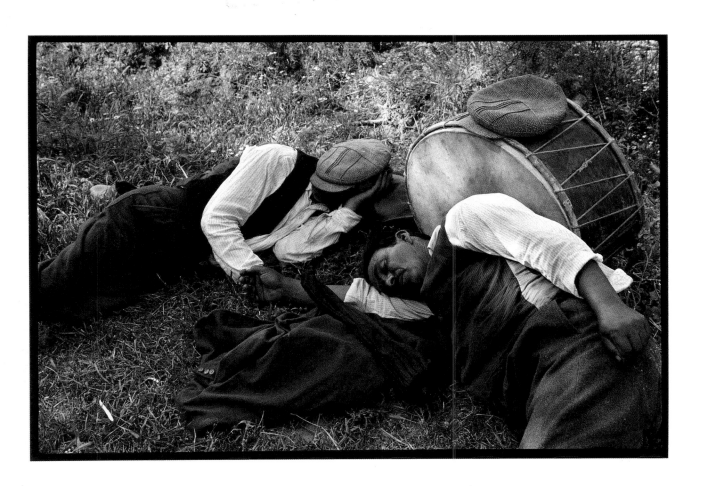

Constantine Manos, Yougoslavia, *Yougoslavie,* Jugoslawien, 1961-1964. **17**

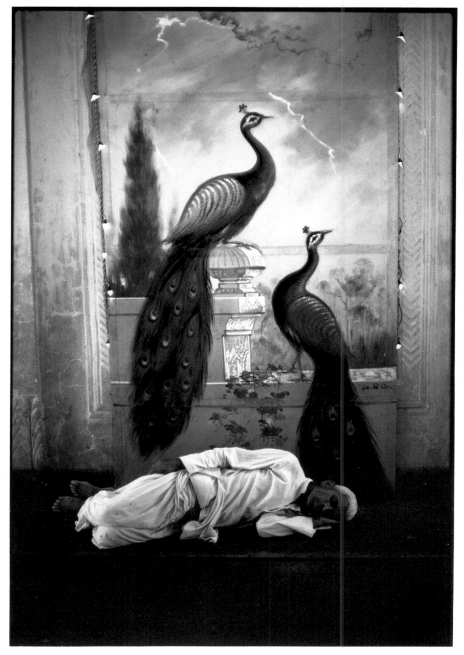

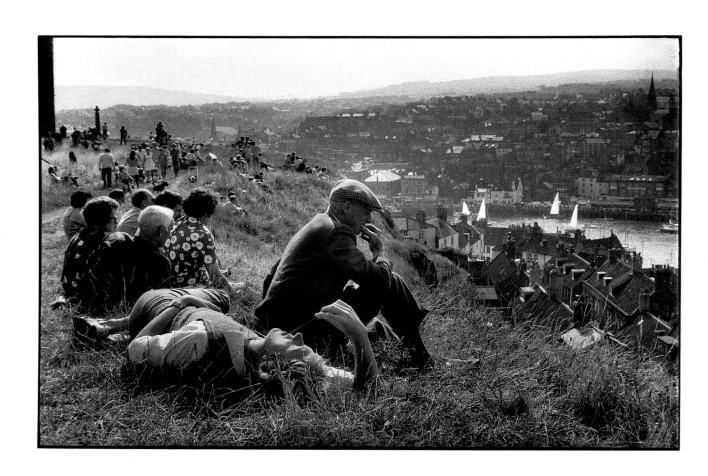

Ian Berry, England, *Angleterre,* England, 1974.

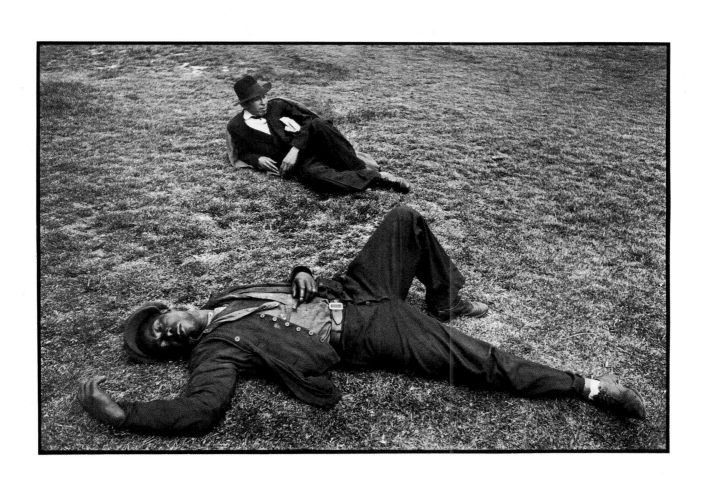

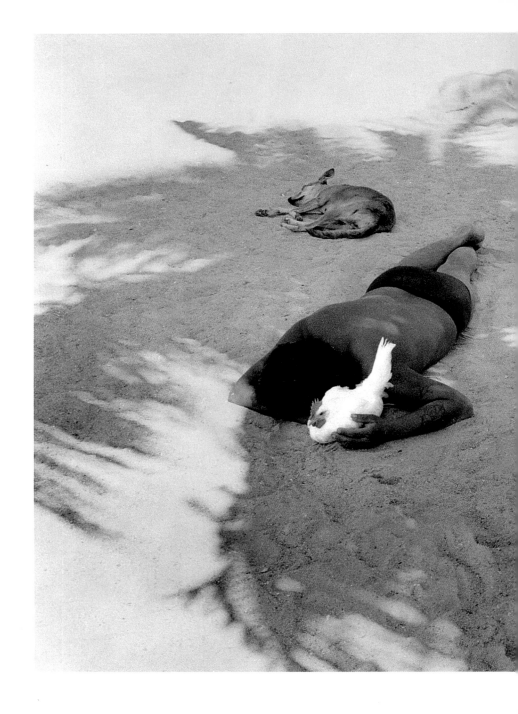

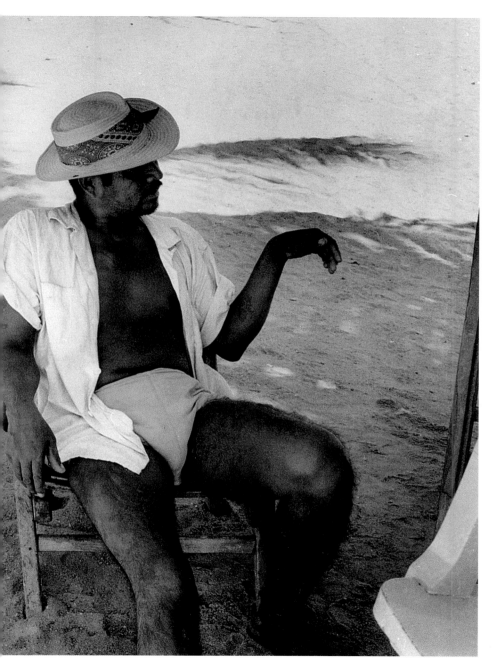

Marc Riboud, Mexico, *Mexique,* Mexiko, 1959. **23**

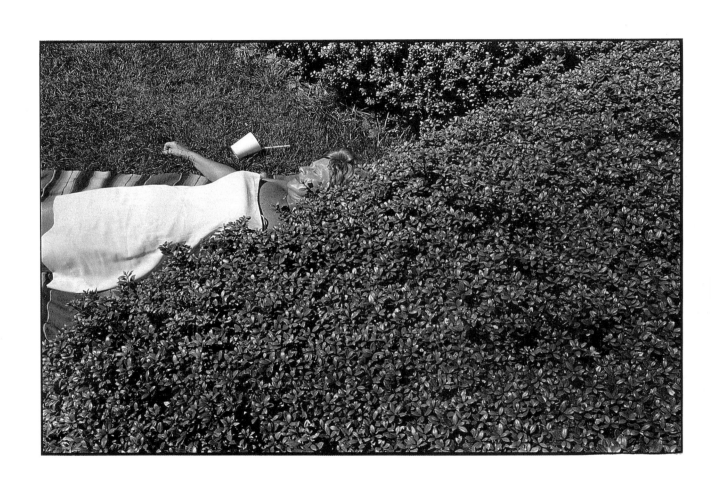

Richard Kalvar, USA, *États-Unis,* USA, 1969.

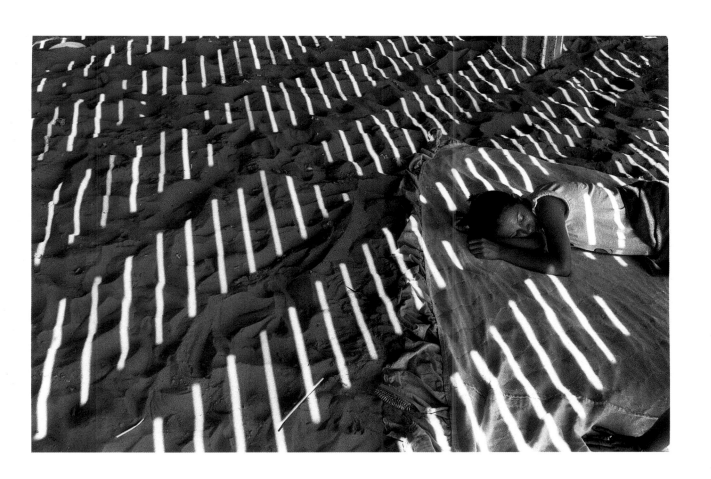

Ferdinando Scianna, USA, *États-Unis,* USA, 1985. **25**

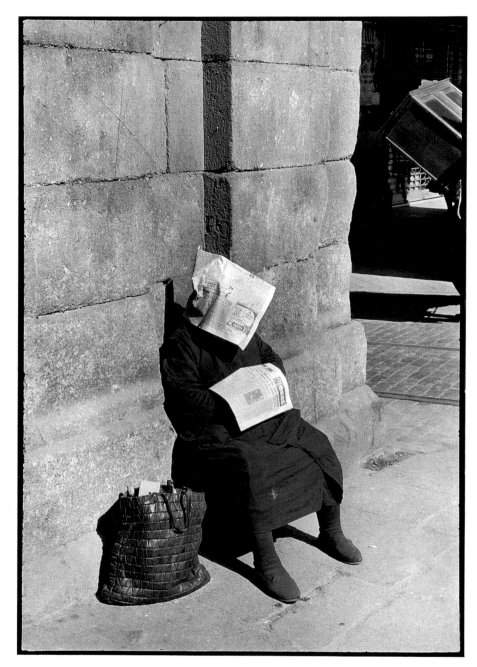

Inge Morath, Spain, *Espagne,* Spanien, 1955.

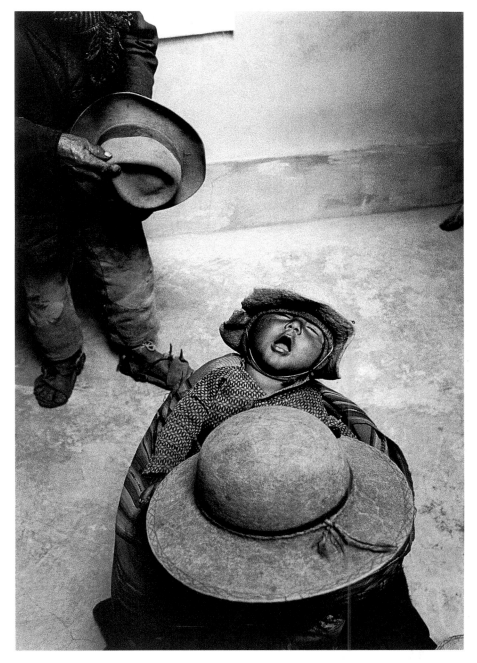

Ferdinando Scianna, Bolivia, *Bolivie,* Bolivien, 1986. **27**

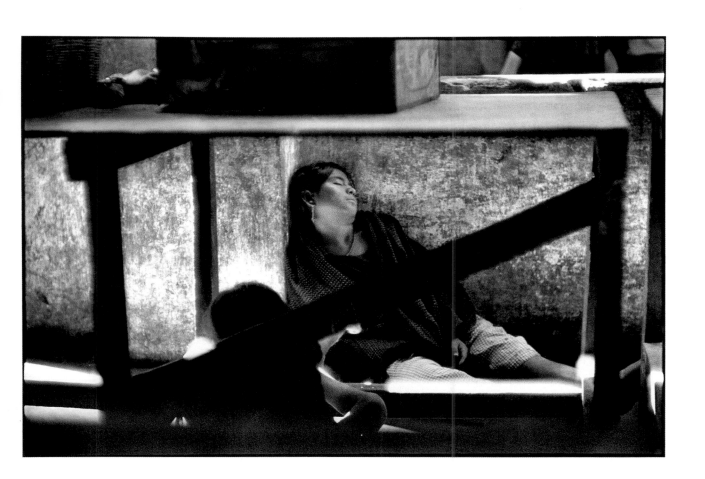

Henri Cartier-Bresson, Mexico, *Mexique,* Mexiko, 1934. **29**

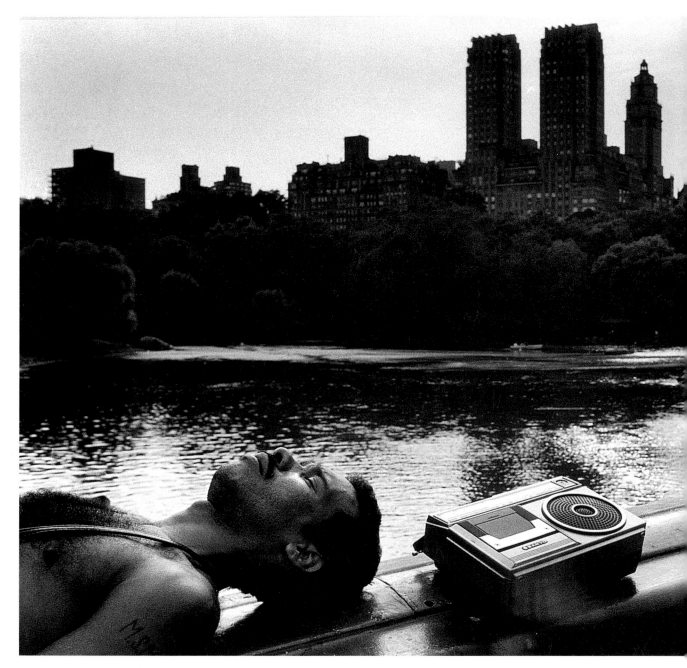

| Ferdinando Scianna, USA, *États-Unis,* USA, 1985.

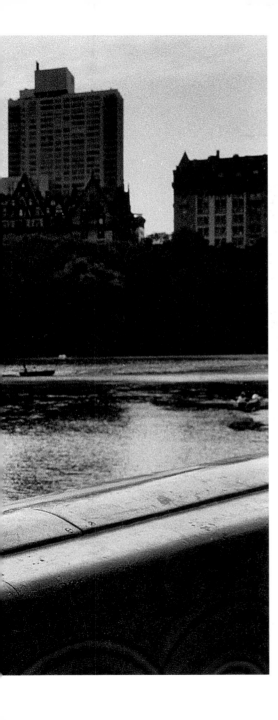

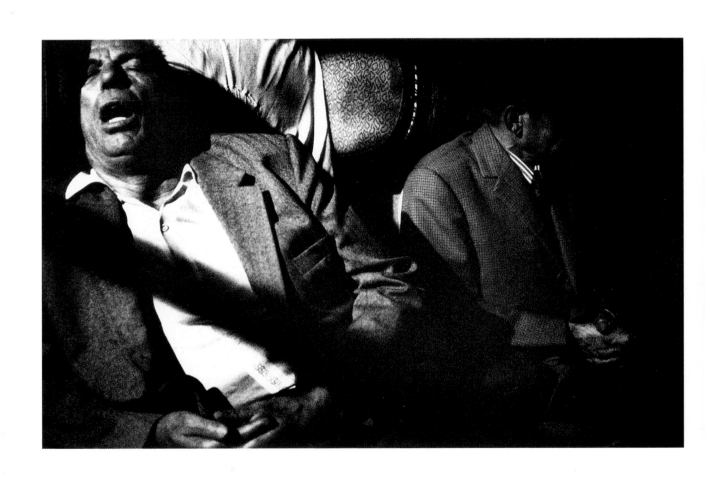

Josef Koudelka, Spain, *Espagne,* Spanien, 1973.

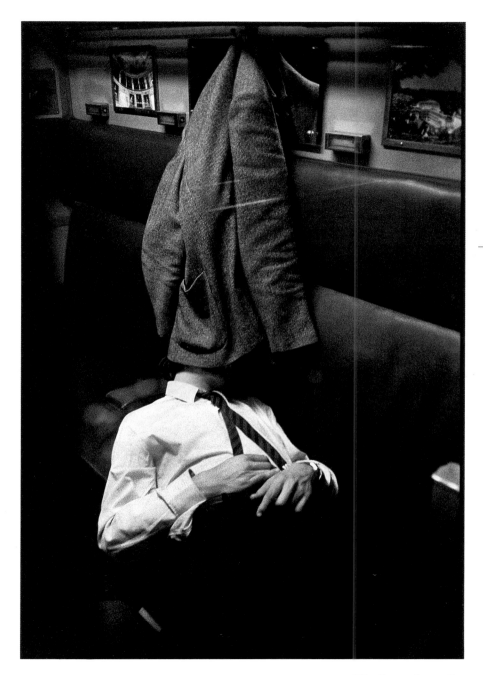

Gilles Peress, France, *France,* Frankreich, 1970. **33**

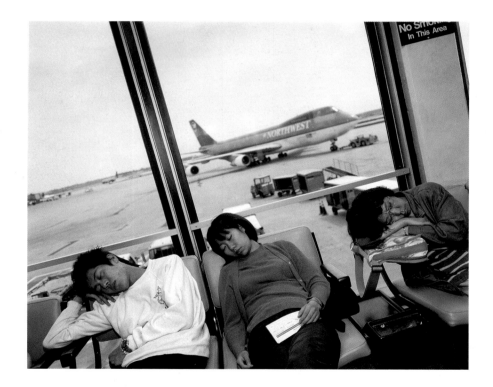

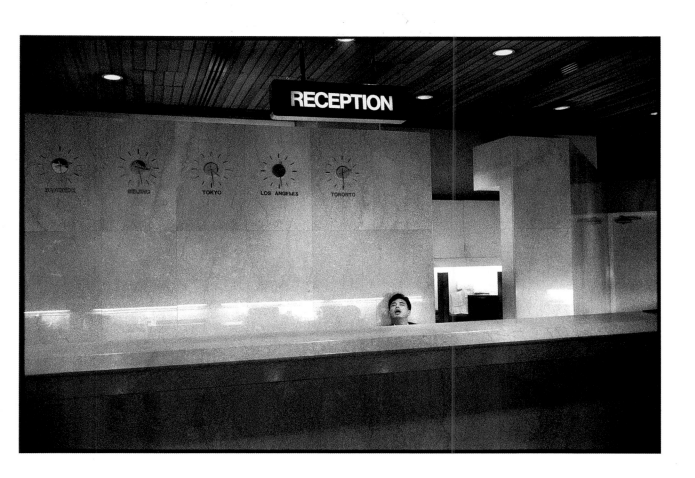

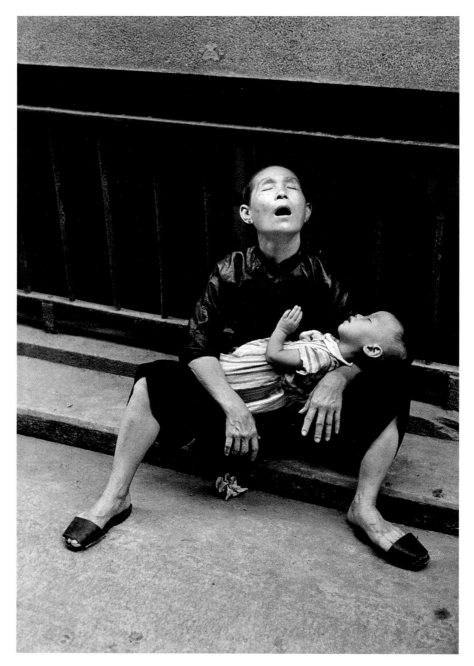

Werner Bischof, Hong Kong, *Hong Kong,* Hongkong, 1952.

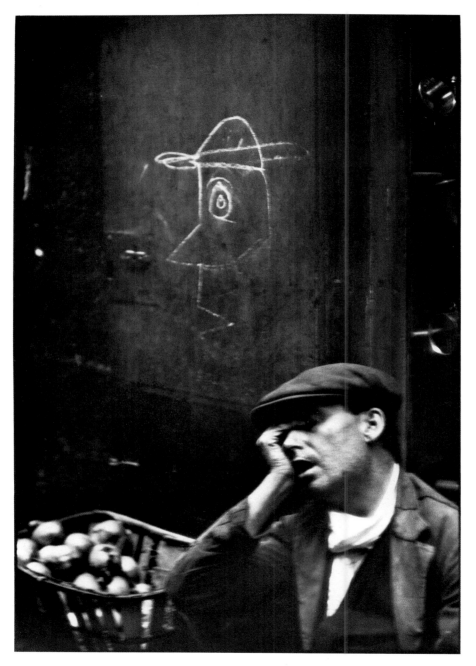

Henri Cartier-Bresson, Spain, *Espagne,* Spanien, 1933. **37**

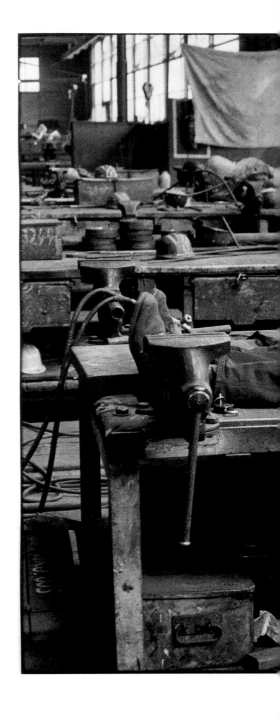

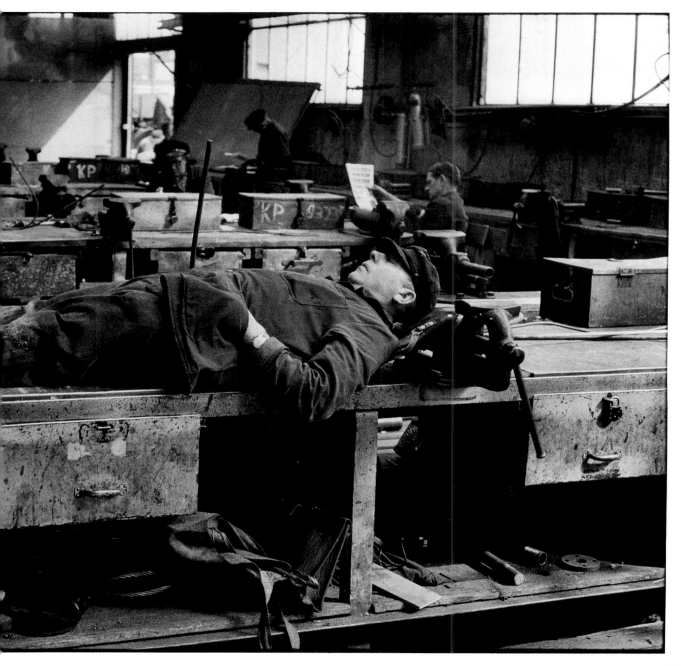

Henri Cartier-Bresson, FRG, *RFA,* BRD, 1962. | **39**

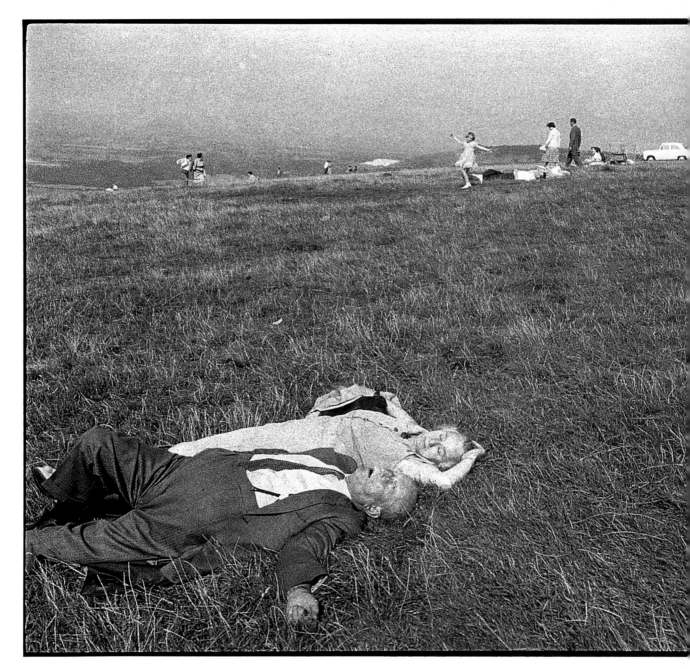

Bruce Davidson, England, *Angleterre,* England, 1960.

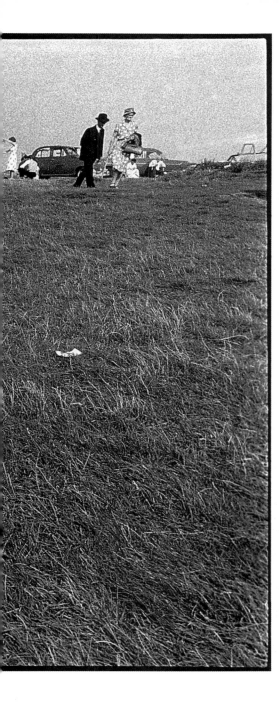

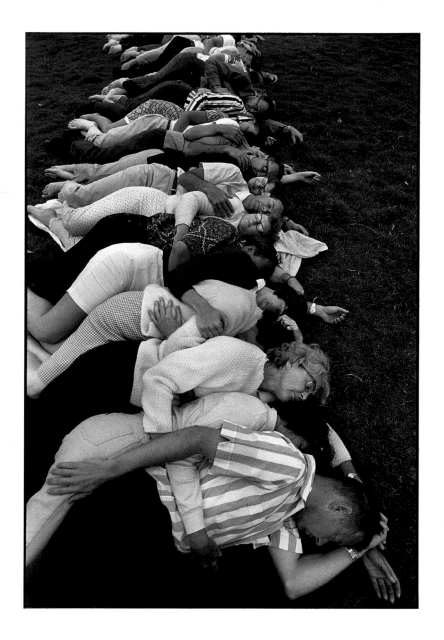

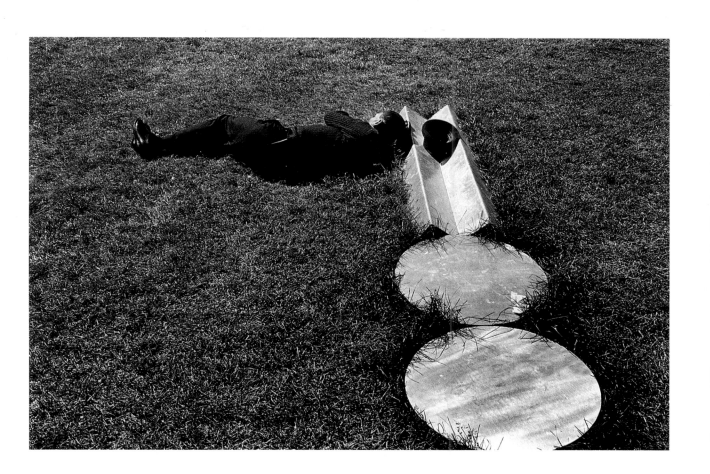

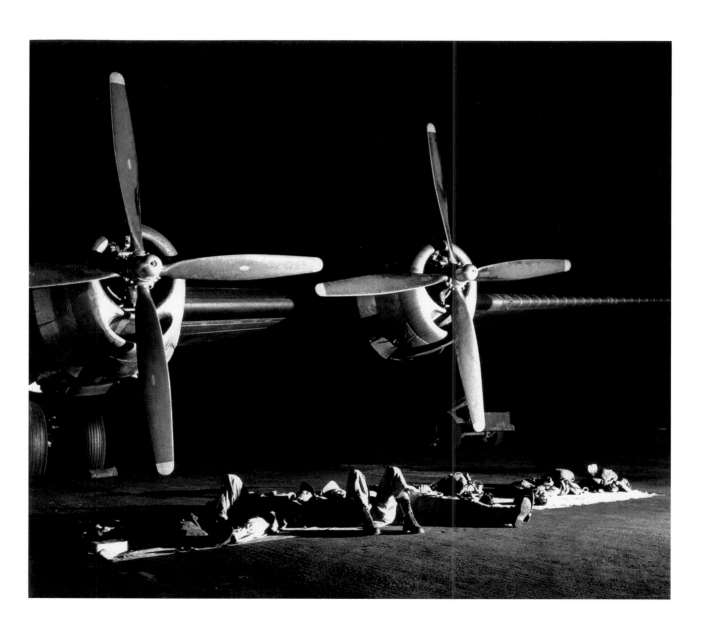

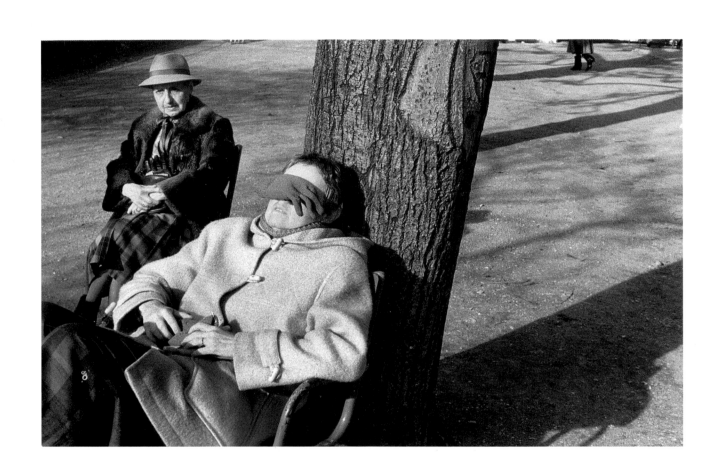

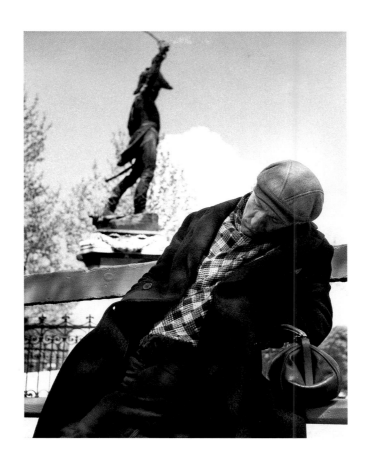

Herbert List, France, *France,* Frankreich, 1936. **47**

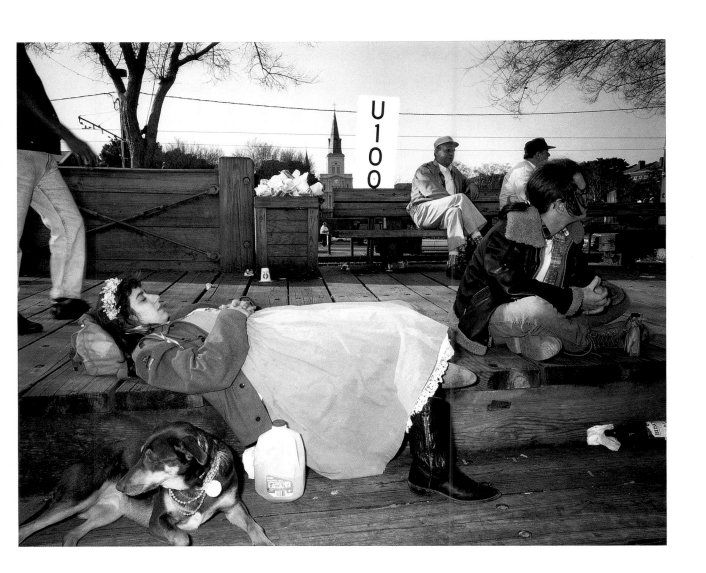

Carl De Keyzer, USA, *États-Unis,* USA, 1990. **49**

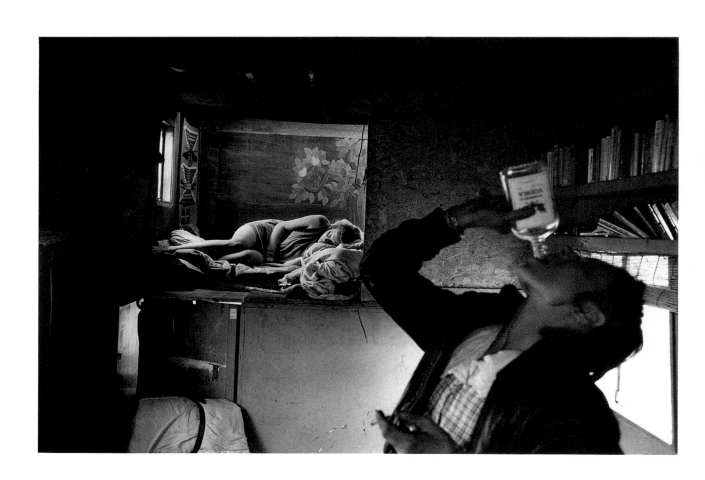

| Donovan Wylie, England, *Angleterre,* England, 1996.

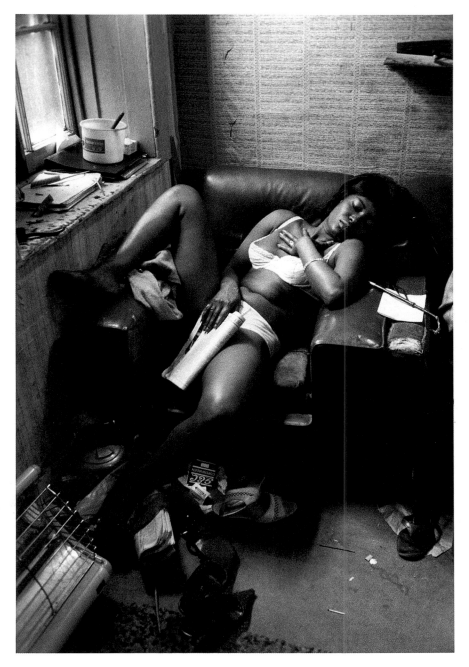

David Hurn, England, *Angleterre,* England, 1965. **51**

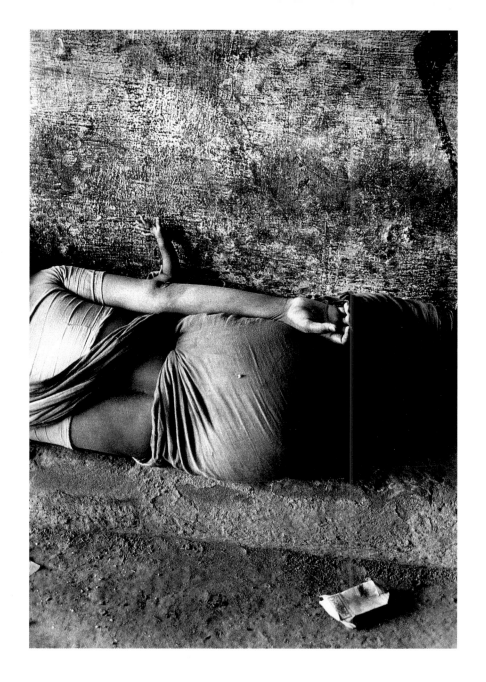

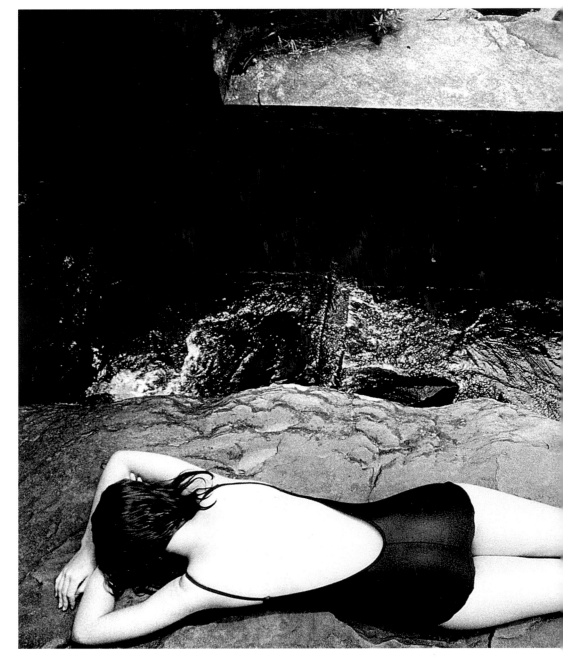

Josef Koudelka, USA, *États-Unis,* USA, 1974.

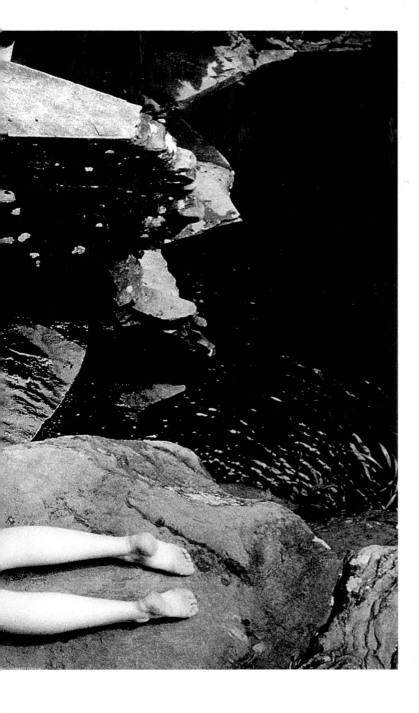

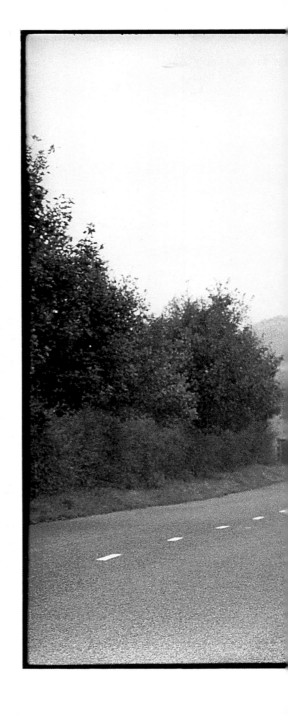

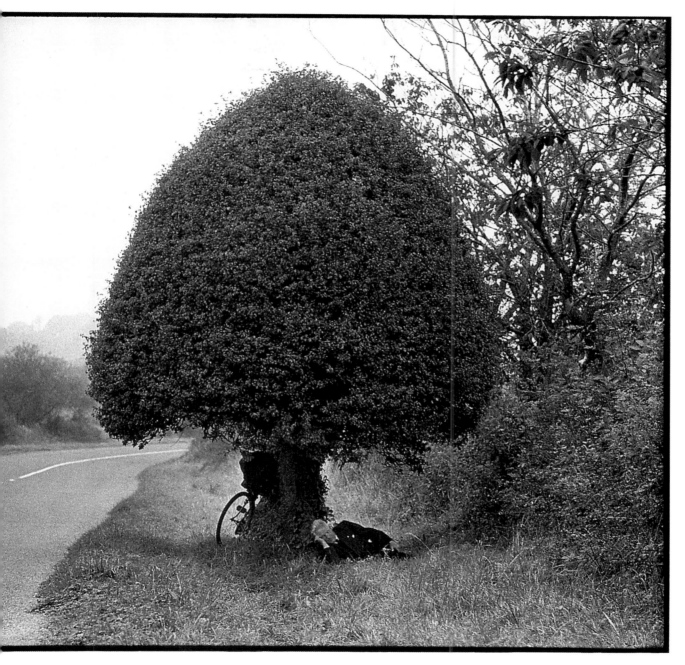

Henri Cartier-Bresson, Ireland, *Irlande, Ireland,* 1962.

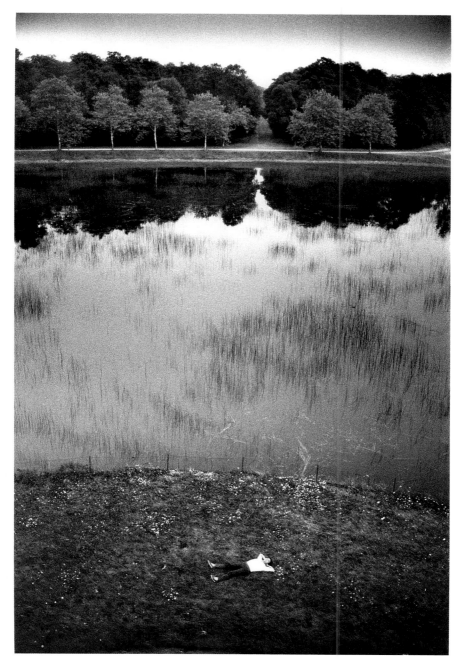

Marc Riboud, France, *France,* Frankreich, 1962.

Spanien.
Inge Morath, 1955.

Page 27: A small child on the shoulders of his father, in a local medical center in Kami, a miners' village in the Andes, Bolivia.
Ferdinando Scianna, 1986.
Page 27 : *Enfant sur les épaules de son père dans un centre médical à Kami, village de mineurs dans les Andes, Bolivie.*
Ferdinando Scianna, 1986.
Seite 27: Kind auf den Schultern seines Vaters in einem medizinischen Versorgungszentrum in Kami. Bergarbeiterdorf der Anden, Bolivien.
Ferdinando Scianna, 1986.

Page 29: Juchitan, Mexico.
Henri Cartier-Bresson, 1934.
Page 29 : *Juchitan, Mexique.*
Henri Cartier-Bresson, 1934.
Seite 29: Juchitan, Mexiko.
Henri Cartier-Bresson, 1934.

Pages 30-31: Central Park, New York City, USA.
Ferdinando Scianna, 1985.
Pages 30-31 : *Central Park, New York, États-Unis.*
Ferdinando Scianna, 1985.
Seite 30-31: Central Park, New York, USA.
Ferdinando Scianna, 1985.

Page 32: Oviedo, Asturias, Spain.
Josef Koudelka, 1973.
Page 32 : *Oviedo, Asturies, Espagne.*
Josef Koudelka, 1973.
Seite 32: Oviedo, Asturias, Spanien.
Josef Koudelka, 1973.

Page 33: France.
Gilles Peress, 1970.
Page 33 : *France.*
Gilles Peress, 1970.
Seite 33: Frankreich.
Gilles Peress, 1970.

Page 34: In the Departure Lounge at Chicago Airport, USA.
Martin Parr, 1997.
Page 34 : *Dans la salle d'embarquement de l'aéroport de Chicago, États-Unis.*
Martin Parr, 1997.
Seite 34: In der Abflughalle des Flugplatzes von Chicago, USA.
Martin Parr, 1997.

Page 35: Hong Kong.
Patrick Zachmann, 1995.
Page 35 : *Hong Kong.*
Patrick Zachmann, 1995.
Seite 35: Hongkong.
Patrick Zachmann, 1995.

Page 36: Afternoon in Hong Kong.
Werner Bischof, 1952.
Page 36 : *Après-midi à Hong Kong.*
Werner Bischof, 1952.
Seite 36: Nachmittags in Hongkong.
Werner Bischof, 1952.

Page 37: Barrio Chino, Barcelona, Spain.
Henri Cartier-Bresson, 1933.
Page 37 : *Barrio Chino, Barcelone, Espagne.*
Henri Cartier-Bresson, 1933.
Seite 37: Barrio Chino, Barcelona, Spanien.
Henri Cartier-Bresson, 1933.

Pages 38-39: Shipyard, lunch hour. Bremen, FRG.

Henri Cartier-Bresson, 1962.
Pages 38-39 : *Chantier naval, pause à l'heure du déjeuner. Brême, RFA.*
Henri Cartier-Bresson, 1962.
Seite 38-39: Schiffswerft, Mittagspause. Bremen, BRD.
Henri Cartier-Bresson, 1962.

Pages 40-41: Hastings, England.
Bruce Davidson, 1960.
Pages 40-41 : *Hastings, Angleterre.*
Bruce Davidson, 1960.
Seite 40-41: Hastings, England.
Bruce Davidson, 1960.

Page 42: Esalin Insitute participants in a body-awareness exercise. Big Sur, California, USA.
Paul Fusco, 1967.
Page 42 : *Des membres de l'institut Esalin en plein exercice d' « éveil du corps ». Big Sur, Californie, États-Unis.*
Paul Fusco, 1967.
Seite 42: Mitglieder des Esalin-Insituts bei der Übung „Erwachen des Körpers". Big Sur, Kalifornien, USA.
Paul Fusco, 1967.

Page 43: Central Park, New York City, USA.
Richard Kalvar, 1969.
Page 43 : *Central Park, New York, États-Unis.*
Richard Kalvar, 1969.
Seite 43: Central Park, New York, USA.
Richard Kalvar, 1969.

Page 45: American Aircrew resting beneath their planes. Okinawa, Japan.
Werner Bischof, 1951.

Page 45 : *Soldats américains se reposant sous leur avion. Okinawa, Japon.*
Werner Bischof, 1951.
Seite 45: Eine sich unter ihrem Flugzeug ausruhende Mannschaft der amerikanischen Luftwaffe. Okinawa, Japan.
Werner Bischof, 1951.

Page 46: February sun in the Luxembourg Gardens, Paris, France.
Marc Riboud, 1985.
Page 46 : *Soleil de février dans le jardin du Luxembourg, Paris, France.*
Marc Riboud, 1985.
Seite 46: Februarsonne im Jardin du Luxembourg, Paris, Frankreich.
Marc Riboud, 1985.

Page 47: Dreaming of the glories of General Ney. Paris, France.
Herbert List, 1936.
Page 47 : *Rêvant à la gloire du général Ney. Paris, France.*
Herbert List, 1936.
Seite 47: Vom Ruhm des Generals Ney träumend. Paris, Frankreich.
Herbert List, 1936.

Page 49: Mardi Gras, New Orleans, Louisiana, USA.
Carl De Keyzer, 1990.
Page 49 : *Mardi Gras à la Nouvelle-Orléans, Louisiane, États-Unis.*
Carl De Keyzer, 1990.
Seite 49: Mardi Gras in New Orleans, Louisiana, USA.
Carl De Keyzer, 1990.

Page 50: Whitechapel Travellers site, London,

England.
Donovan Wylie, 1996.
Page 50 : *Whitechapel
Travellers, Londres, Angleterre.
Donovan Wylie, 1996.*
Seite 50: Whitechapel
Travellers, London, England.
Donovan Wylie, 1996.

■ **Page 51:** Soho, London,
England.
David Hurn, 1965.
Page 51 : *Dans le quartier de
Soho, Londres, Angleterre.
David Hurn, 1965.*
Seite 51: Im Soho-Viertel,
London, England.
David Hurn, 1965.

■ **Page 53:** Sidewalk in Calcutta,
India.
Raghu Rai, 1989.
Page 53 : *Trottoir de Calcutta,
Inde.
Raghu Rai, 1989.*
Seite 53: Trottoir in Calcutta,
Indien.
Raghu Rai, 1989.

■ **Pages 54-55:** USA.
Josef Koudelka, 1974.
Pages 54-55 : *États-Unis.
Josef Koudelka, 1974.*
Seite 54-55: USA.
Josef Koudelka, 1974.

■ **Pages 56-57:** County Cork,
province of Munster, Ireland.
Henri Cartier-Bresson, 1962.
Pages 56-57 : *Comté de
Cork, province de Munster,
Irlande.
Henri Cartier-Bresson, 1962.*
Seite 56-57: Grafschaft Cork,
Provinz Munster, Irland.
Henri Cartier-Bresson, 1962.

■ **Page 59:** The photographer
William Klein at the edge of
the Chanteloup Pagoda pond
near Amboise, France.
Marc Riboud, 1962.
Page 59 : *Le photographe
William Klein au bord de
l'étang de la Pagode de
Chanteloup, près d'Amboise,
France.
Marc Riboud, 1962.*
Seite 59: Der Fotograf
William Klein am Teich der
Pagode von Chanteloup in der
Nähe von Amboise,
Frankreich.
Marc Riboud, 1962.